# This Essential Oils Journal Belongs To:

©2019 Paislee Paperie. All rights reserved.
No part of this book may be reproduced without written permission of the copyright owner, except for the use of limited quotations for the purpose of book reviews.

# Essential Oil Inventory

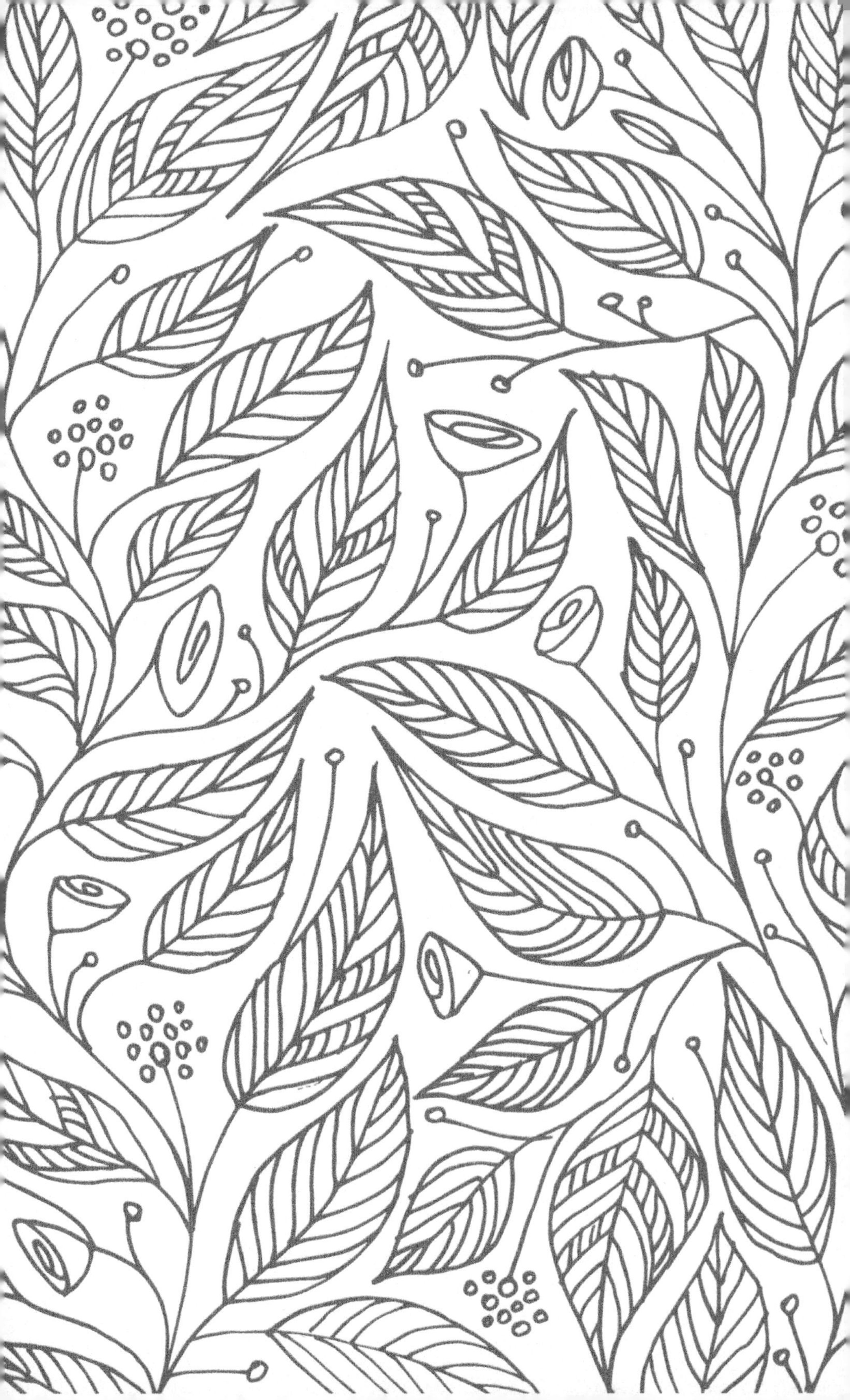

# Essential Oil Inventory

| NAME | USED FOR | DATE OPENED | FAVORITE? |
|------|----------|-------------|-----------|
|      |          |             |           |

# Essential Oil Inventory

| NAME | USED FOR | DATE OPENED | FAVORITE? |
|------|----------|-------------|-----------|
|      |          |             |           |

# Essential Oil Inventory

| NAME | USED FOR | DATE OPENED | FAVORITE? |
|------|----------|-------------|-----------|
|      |          |             |           |

# Essential Oil Inventory

| NAME | USED FOR | DATE OPENED | FAVORITE? |
| --- | --- | --- | --- |
| | | | |

# Essential Oil Inventory

| NAME | USED FOR | DATE OPENED | FAVORITE? |
| --- | --- | --- | --- |
| | | | |

# Essential Oil Inventory

| NAME | USED FOR | DATE OPENED | FAVORITE? |
| --- | --- | --- | --- |
| | | | |

# Essential Oil Wish List

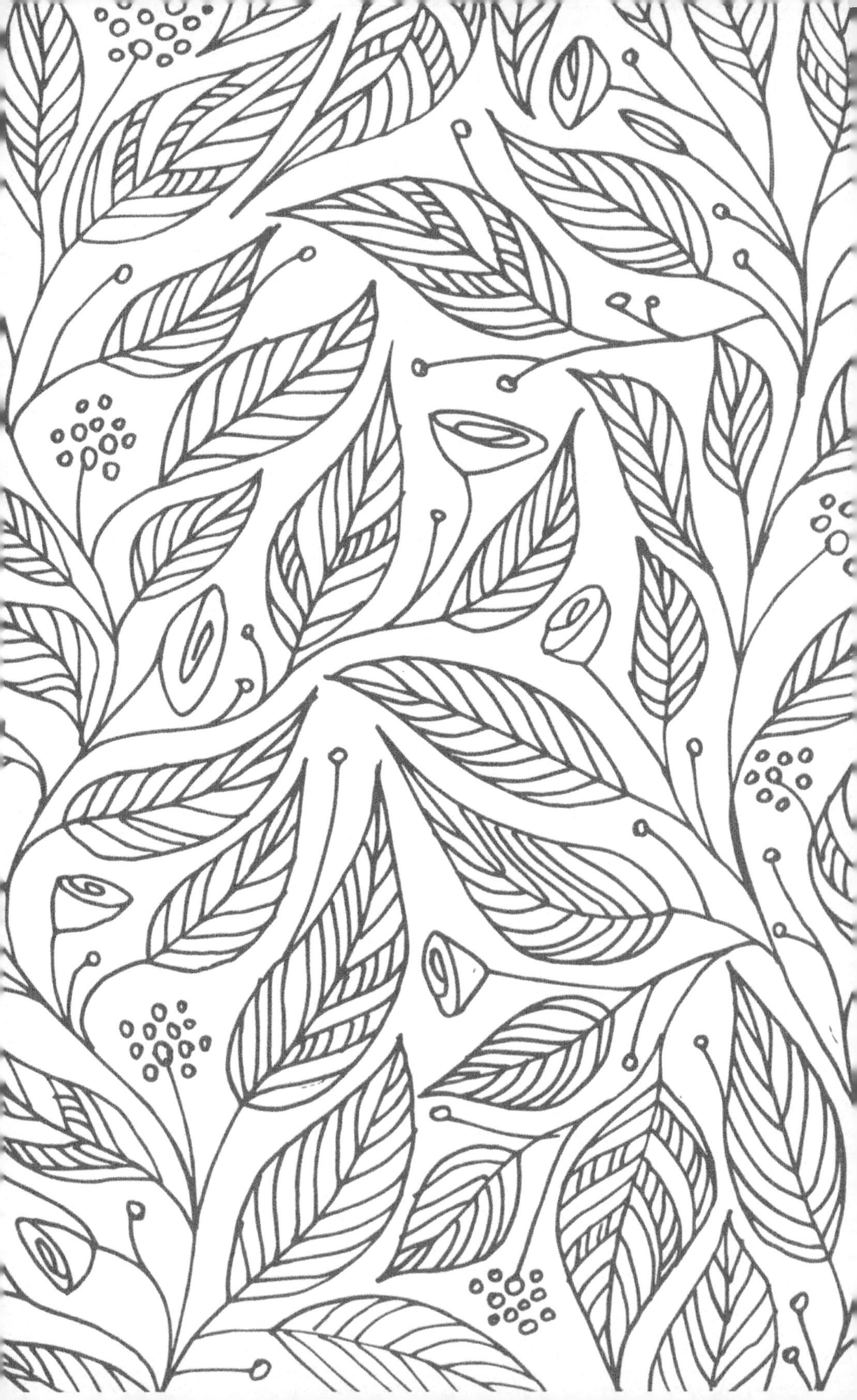

# Essential Oil Wish List

| NAME | USED FOR | PRICE | KID SAFE? |
|------|----------|-------|-----------|
|      |          |       |           |

# Essential Oil Wish List

| NAME | USED FOR | PRICE | KID SAFE? |
| --- | --- | --- | --- |
|  |  |  |  |
|  |  |  |  |
|  |  |  |  |
|  |  |  |  |
|  |  |  |  |
|  |  |  |  |
|  |  |  |  |
|  |  |  |  |
|  |  |  |  |
|  |  |  |  |
|  |  |  |  |
|  |  |  |  |
|  |  |  |  |

# Essential Oil Wish List

| NAME | USED FOR | PRICE | KID SAFE? |
| --- | --- | --- | --- |

# Essential Oil Wish List

| NAME | USED FOR | PRICE | KID SAFE? |
|------|----------|-------|-----------|
|      |          |       |           |

# Essential Oil Wish List

| NAME | USED FOR | PRICE | KID SAFE? |
| --- | --- | --- | --- |

# Essential Oil Wish List

| NAME | USED FOR | PRICE | KID SAFE? |
| --- | --- | --- | --- |

# My Oil Ratings

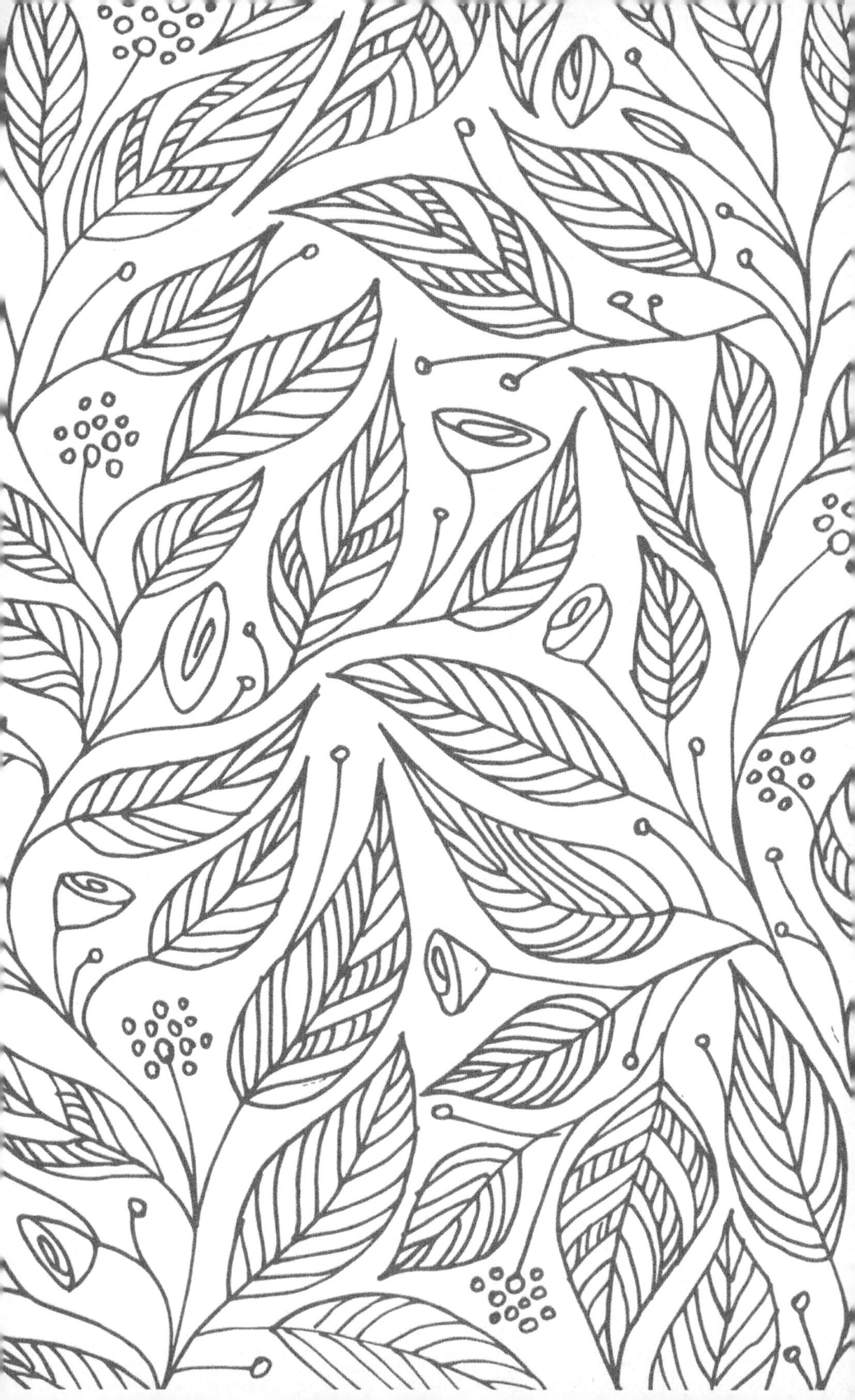

# My Oil Ratings

**PURPOSE OF OIL**

NAME:

MY RATING:

**PURPOSE OF OIL**

NAME:

MY RATING:

**PURPOSE OF OIL**

NAME:

MY RATING:

**PURPOSE OF OIL**

NAME:

MY RATING:

**PURPOSE OF OIL**

NAME:

MY RATING:

**NOTES:**

# My Oil Ratings

**PURPOSE OF OIL**

NAME:

MY RATING:

**PURPOSE OF OIL**

NAME:

MY RATING:

**PURPOSE OF OIL**

NAME:

MY RATING:

**PURPOSE OF OIL**

NAME:

MY RATING:

**PURPOSE OF OIL**

NAME:

MY RATING:

**NOTES:**

# My Oil Ratings

**PURPOSE OF OIL**

NAME:

MY RATING:

**PURPOSE OF OIL**

NAME:

MY RATING:

**PURPOSE OF OIL**

NAME:

MY RATING:

**PURPOSE OF OIL**

NAME:

MY RATING:

**PURPOSE OF OIL**

NAME:

MY RATING:

**NOTES:**

# My Oil Ratings

**PURPOSE OF OIL**

NAME:

MY RATING:

**PURPOSE OF OIL**

NAME:

MY RATING:

**PURPOSE OF OIL**

NAME:

MY RATING:

**PURPOSE OF OIL**

NAME:

MY RATING:

**PURPOSE OF OIL**

NAME:

MY RATING:

**NOTES:**

# My Oil Ratings

**PURPOSE OF OIL**

NAME:

MY RATING:

**PURPOSE OF OIL**

NAME:

MY RATING:

**PURPOSE OF OIL**

NAME:

MY RATING:

**PURPOSE OF OIL**

NAME:

MY RATING:

**PURPOSE OF OIL**

NAME:

MY RATING:

**NOTES:**

# My Oil Ratings

**PURPOSE OF OIL**

NAME:

MY RATING:

**PURPOSE OF OIL**

NAME:

MY RATING:

**PURPOSE OF OIL**

NAME:

MY RATING:

**PURPOSE OF OIL**

NAME:

MY RATING:

**PURPOSE OF OIL**

NAME:

MY RATING:

**NOTES:**

# My Oil Ratings

**PURPOSE OF OIL**

NAME:

MY RATING:

**PURPOSE OF OIL**

NAME:

MY RATING:

**PURPOSE OF OIL**

NAME:

MY RATING:

**PURPOSE OF OIL**

NAME:

MY RATING:

**PURPOSE OF OIL**

NAME:

MY RATING:

**NOTES:**

# My Oil Ratings

**PURPOSE OF OIL**

NAME:

MY RATING:

**PURPOSE OF OIL**

NAME:

MY RATING:

**PURPOSE OF OIL**

NAME:

MY RATING:

**PURPOSE OF OIL**

NAME:

MY RATING:

**PURPOSE OF OIL**

NAME:

MY RATING:

**NOTES:**

# My Oil Ratings

**PURPOSE OF OIL**

NAME:

MY RATING:

**PURPOSE OF OIL**

NAME:

MY RATING:

**PURPOSE OF OIL**

NAME:

MY RATING:

**PURPOSE OF OIL**

NAME:

MY RATING:

**PURPOSE OF OIL**

NAME:

MY RATING:

**NOTES:**

# My Oil Ratings

**PURPOSE OF OIL**

NAME:

MY RATING:

**PURPOSE OF OIL**

NAME:

MY RATING:

**PURPOSE OF OIL**

NAME:

MY RATING:

**PURPOSE OF OIL**

NAME:

MY RATING:

**PURPOSE OF OIL**

NAME:

MY RATING:

**NOTES:**

# My Favorite Oils

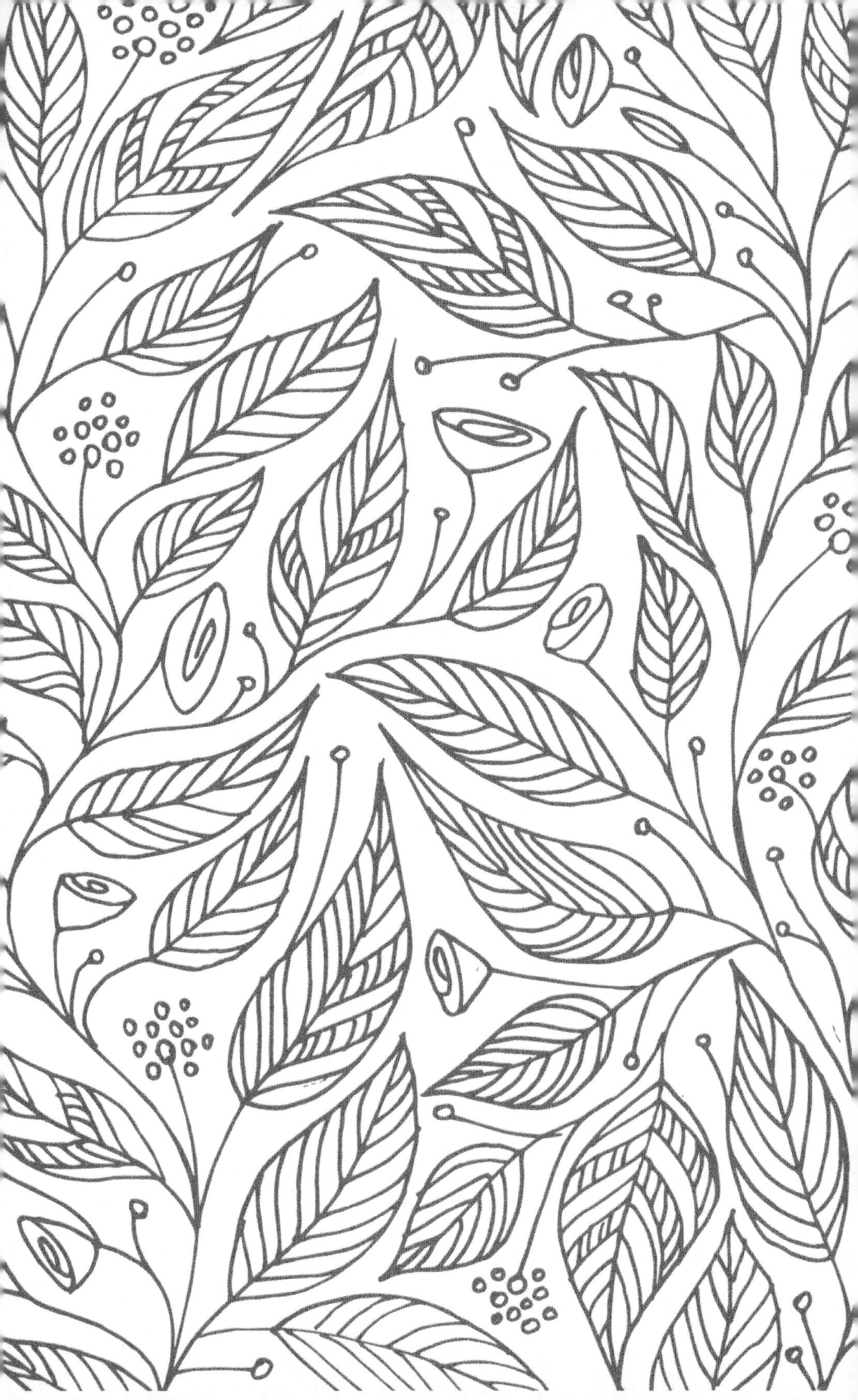

# My Favorite Oils

ENERGY

CALMING

SLEEP

FOCUS/CLARITY

WELLNESS

ROMANCE

ANXIETY

JOYFUL

# My Favorite Oils

**MORNING**

**IMMUNE**

**UPLIFTING**

**BEDTIME**

**BATHS**

**WOMEN**

**MEN**

**KIDS**

# My Favorite Blends

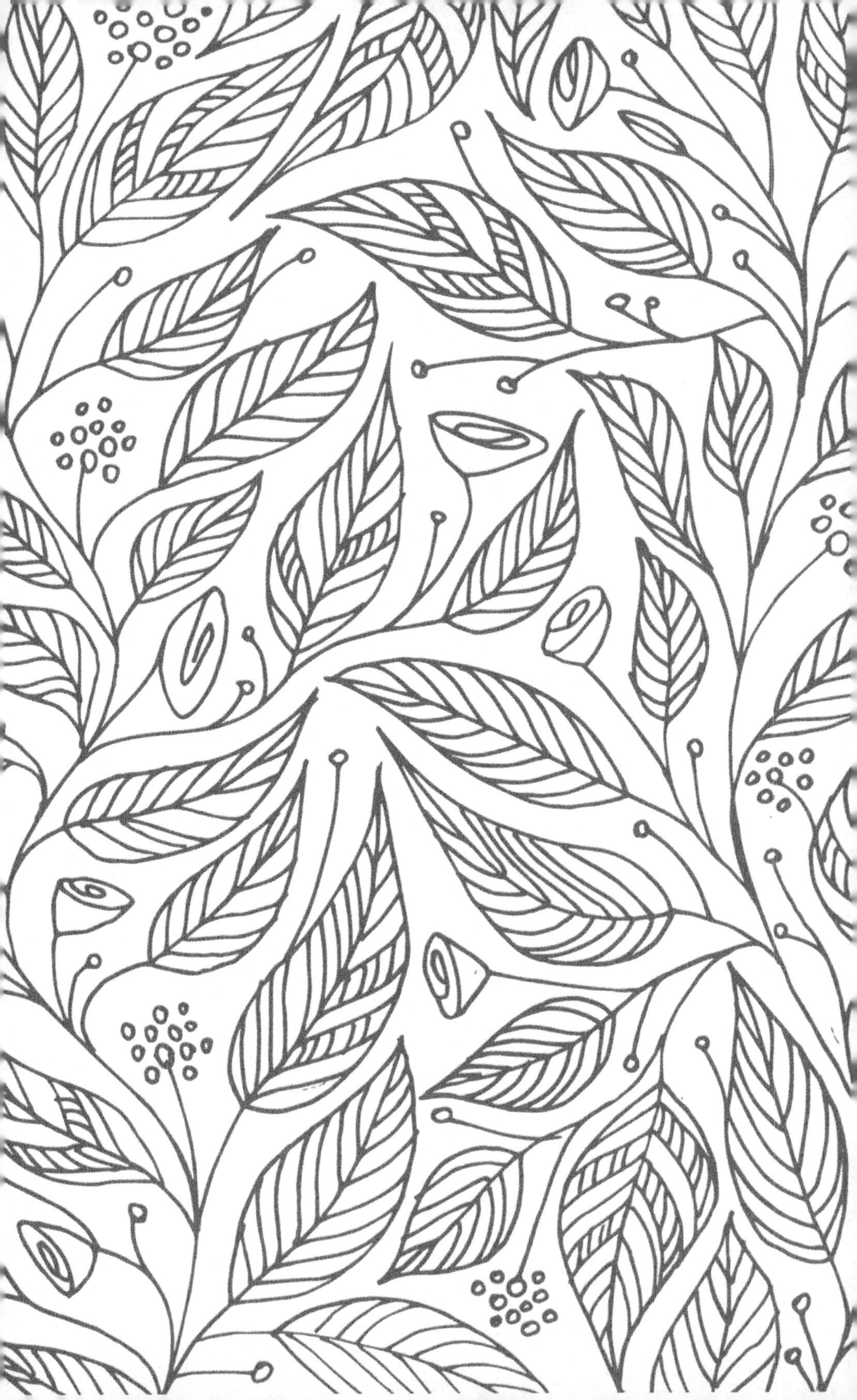

# My Favorite Blends

NAME: USED FOR:

**INGREDIENTS:**

NOTES:

NAME: USED FOR:

**INGREDIENTS:**

NOTES:

# My Favorite Blends

NAME:                                                USED FOR:

**INGREDIENTS:**

NOTES:

---

NAME:                                                USED FOR:

**INGREDIENTS:**

NOTES:

# My Favorite Blends

NAME: USED FOR:

**INGREDIENTS:**

NOTES:

NAME: USED FOR:

**INGREDIENTS:**

NOTES:

# My Favorite Blends

NAME:                                              USED FOR:

**INGREDIENTS:**

NOTES:

---

NAME:                                              USED FOR:

**INGREDIENTS:**

NOTES:

# My Favorite Blends

NAME:                                                USED FOR:

**INGREDIENTS:**

NOTES:

---

NAME:                                                USED FOR:

**INGREDIENTS:**

NOTES:

# My Favorite Blends

NAME: USED FOR:

**INGREDIENTS:**

NOTES:

NAME: USED FOR:

**INGREDIENTS:**

NOTES:

# My Favorite Blends

NAME: USED FOR:

**INGREDIENTS:**

NOTES:

NAME: USED FOR:

**INGREDIENTS:**

NOTES:

# My Favorite Blends

NAME:  USED FOR:

**INGREDIENTS:**

NOTES:

NAME:  USED FOR:

**INGREDIENTS:**

NOTES:

# My Favorite Blends

NAME:  USED FOR:

**INGREDIENTS:**

NOTES:

NAME:  USED FOR:

**INGREDIENTS:**

NOTES:

# My Favorite Blends

NAME: USED FOR:

**INGREDIENTS:**

NOTES:

NAME: USED FOR:

**INGREDIENTS:**

NOTES:

# My Favorite Blends

NAME:  USED FOR:

**INGREDIENTS:**

NOTES:

---

NAME:  USED FOR:

**INGREDIENTS:**

NOTES:

# My Favorite Blends

NAME:

USED FOR:

**INGREDIENTS:**

NOTES:

NAME:

USED FOR:

**INGREDIENTS:**

NOTES:

# My Essential Oil Recipes

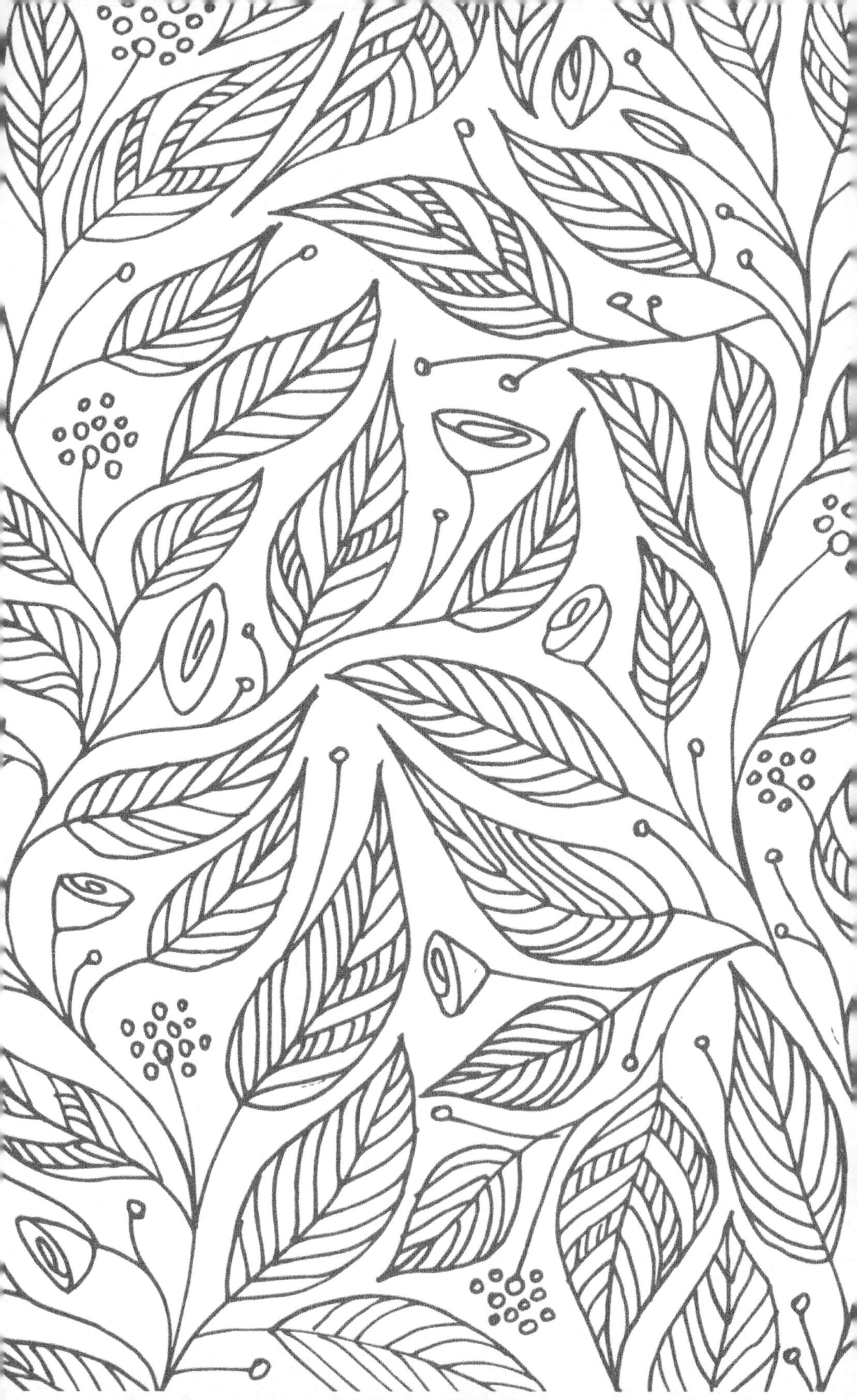

# Essential Oil Recipes

NAME:

OILS USED:

USED FOR:

INSTRUCTIONS:

## Aromatic
- ◯ DIFFUSE
- ◯ INHALE
- ◯ SPRAY BOTTLE
- ◯

## Topical
- ◯ DILLUTE
- ◯ NEAT
- ◯ TEMPLE
- ◯ CHEST
- ◯ STOMACH
- ◯ FEET
- ◯

## Internal
- ◯ ADD TO DRINKING WATER
- ◯ ADD IN FOOD
- ◯ ADD IN CAPSULE
- ◯ UNDER TONGUE
- ◯

NOTES:

# Essential Oil Recipes

NAME:

OILS USED:

USED FOR:

INSTRUCTIONS:

## Aromatic
- ○ DIFFUSE
- ○ INHALE
- ○ SPRAY BOTTLE
- ○ _____

## Topical
- ○ DILLUTE
- ○ NEAT
- ○ TEMPLE
- ○ CHEST
- ○ STOMACH
- ○ FEET
- ○ _____

## Internal
- ○ ADD TO DRINKING WATER
- ○ ADD IN FOOD
- ○ ADD IN CAPSULE
- ○ UNDER TONGUE
- ○ _____

NOTES:

# Essential Oil Recipes

NAME: _____

OILS USED: _____

USED FOR: _____
_____

INSTRUCTIONS: _____
_____
_____
_____

## Aromatic
- ◯ DIFFUSE
- ◯ INHALE
- ◯ SPRAY BOTTLE
- ◯ _____

## Topical
- ◯ DILLUTE
- ◯ NEAT
- ◯ TEMPLE
- ◯ CHEST
- ◯ STOMACH
- ◯ FEET
- ◯ _____

## Internal
- ◯ ADD TO DRINKING WATER
- ◯ ADD IN FOOD
- ◯ ADD IN CAPSULE
- ◯ UNDER TONGUE
- ◯ _____

NOTES:
_____
_____

# Essential Oil Recipes

NAME:

OILS USED:

USED FOR:

INSTRUCTIONS:

## Aromatic
- ◯ DIFFUSE
- ◯ INHALE
- ◯ SPRAY BOTTLE
- ◯ _____

## Topical
- ◯ DILLUTE
- ◯ NEAT
- ◯ TEMPLE
- ◯ CHEST
- ◯ STOMACH
- ◯ FEET
- ◯ _____

## Internal
- ◯ ADD TO DRINKING WATER
- ◯ ADD IN FOOD
- ◯ ADD IN CAPSULE
- ◯ UNDER TONGUE
- ◯ _____

NOTES:

# Essential Oil Recipes

NAME: _____

OILS USED: _____

USED FOR: _____
_____

INSTRUCTIONS: _____
_____
_____

### Aromatic
- ◯ DIFFUSE
- ◯ INHALE
- ◯ SPRAY BOTTLE
- ◯ _____

### Topical
- ◯ DILLUTE
- ◯ NEAT
- ◯ TEMPLE
- ◯ CHEST
- ◯ STOMACH
- ◯ FEET
- ◯ _____

### Internal
- ◯ ADD TO DRINKING WATER
- ◯ ADD IN FOOD
- ◯ ADD IN CAPSULE
- ◯ UNDER TONGUE
- ◯ _____

NOTES: _____
_____
_____

# Essential Oil Recipes

NAME:

OILS USED:

USED FOR:

INSTRUCTIONS:

## Aromatic
- ◯ DIFFUSE
- ◯ INHALE
- ◯ SPRAY BOTTLE
- ◯

## Topical
- ◯ DILLUTE
- ◯ NEAT
- ◯ TEMPLE
- ◯ CHEST
- ◯ STOMACH
- ◯ FEET
- ◯

## Internal
- ◯ ADD TO DRINKING WATER
- ◯ ADD IN FOOD
- ◯ ADD IN CAPSULE
- ◯ UNDER TONGUE
- ◯

NOTES:

# Essential Oil Recipes

NAME:

OILS USED:

USED FOR:

INSTRUCTIONS:

## Aromatic
- ◯ DIFFUSE
- ◯ INHALE
- ◯ SPRAY BOTTLE
- ◯ _____

## Topical
- ◯ DILLUTE
- ◯ NEAT
- ◯ TEMPLE
- ◯ CHEST
- ◯ STOMACH
- ◯ FEET
- ◯ _____

## Internal
- ◯ ADD TO DRINKING WATER
- ◯ ADD IN FOOD
- ◯ ADD IN CAPSULE
- ◯ UNDER TONGUE
- ◯ _____

NOTES:

# Essential Oil Recipes

NAME: _____

OILS USED: _____

USED FOR: _____
_____

INSTRUCTIONS: _____
_____
_____
_____

## Aromatic
- ○ DIFFUSE
- ○ INHALE
- ○ SPRAY BOTTLE
- ○ _____

## Topical
- ○ DILLUTE
- ○ NEAT
- ○ TEMPLE
- ○ CHEST
- ○ STOMACH
- ○ FEET
- ○ _____

## Internal
- ○ ADD TO DRINKING WATER
- ○ ADD IN FOOD
- ○ ADD IN CAPSULE
- ○ UNDER TONGUE
- ○ _____

NOTES: _____
_____
_____

# Essential Oil Recipes

NAME: _____

OILS USED: _____

USED FOR: _____
_____

INSTRUCTIONS: _____
_____
_____
_____

## Aromatic
- ○ DIFFUSE
- ○ INHALE
- ○ SPRAY BOTTLE
- ○ _____

## Topical
- ○ DILLUTE
- ○ NEAT
- ○ TEMPLE
- ○ CHEST
- ○ STOMACH
- ○ FEET
- ○ _____

## Internal
- ○ ADD TO DRINKING WATER
- ○ ADD IN FOOD
- ○ ADD IN CAPSULE
- ○ UNDER TONGUE
- ○ _____

NOTES: _____
_____
_____

# Essential Oil Recipes

NAME: _____

OILS USED: _____

USED FOR: _____
_____

INSTRUCTIONS: _____
_____
_____
_____

## Aromatic
- ◯ DIFFUSE
- ◯ INHALE
- ◯ SPRAY BOTTLE
- ◯ _____

## Topical
- ◯ DILLUTE
- ◯ NEAT
- ◯ TEMPLE
- ◯ CHEST
- ◯ STOMACH
- ◯ FEET
- ◯

## Internal
- ◯ ADD TO DRINKING WATER
- ◯ ADD IN FOOD
- ◯ ADD IN CAPSULE
- ◯ UNDER TONGUE
- ◯

NOTES: _____
_____
_____

# Essential Oil Recipes

NAME:

OILS USED:

USED FOR:

INSTRUCTIONS:

## Aromatic
- ◯ DIFFUSE
- ◯ INHALE
- ◯ SPRAY BOTTLE
- ◯

## Topical
- ◯ DILLUTE
- ◯ NEAT
- ◯ TEMPLE
- ◯ CHEST
- ◯ STOMACH
- ◯ FEET
- ◯

## Internal
- ◯ ADD TO DRINKING WATER
- ◯ ADD IN FOOD
- ◯ ADD IN CAPSULE
- ◯ UNDER TONGUE
- ◯

NOTES:

# Essential Oil Recipes

NAME: _____

OILS USED: _____

USED FOR: _____
_____

INSTRUCTIONS: _____
_____
_____
_____

## Aromatic
- ◯ DIFFUSE
- ◯ INHALE
- ◯ SPRAY BOTTLE
- ◯ _____

## Topical
- ◯ DILLUTE
- ◯ NEAT
- ◯ TEMPLE
- ◯ CHEST
- ◯ STOMACH
- ◯ FEET
- ◯ _____

## Internal
- ◯ ADD TO DRINKING WATER
- ◯ ADD IN FOOD
- ◯ ADD IN CAPSULE
- ◯ UNDER TONGUE
- ◯ _____

NOTES: _____
_____
_____

# Essential Oil Recipes

NAME:

OILS USED:

USED FOR:

INSTRUCTIONS:

## Aromatic
- ○ DIFFUSE
- ○ INHALE
- ○ SPRAY BOTTLE
- ○

## Topical
- ○ DILLUTE
- ○ NEAT
- ○ TEMPLE
- ○ CHEST
- ○ STOMACH
- ○ FEET
- ○

## Internal
- ○ ADD TO DRINKING WATER
- ○ ADD IN FOOD
- ○ ADD IN CAPSULE
- ○ UNDER TONGUE
- ○

NOTES:

# Essential Oil Recipes

NAME:

OILS USED:

USED FOR:

INSTRUCTIONS:

## Aromatic
- ○ DIFFUSE
- ○ INHALE
- ○ SPRAY BOTTLE
- ○ 

## Topical
- ○ DILLUTE
- ○ NEAT
- ○ TEMPLE
- ○ CHEST
- ○ STOMACH
- ○ FEET
- ○ 

## Internal
- ○ ADD TO DRINKING WATER
- ○ ADD IN FOOD
- ○ ADD IN CAPSULE
- ○ UNDER TONGUE
- ○ 

NOTES:

# Essential Oil Recipes

NAME:

OILS USED:

USED FOR:


INSTRUCTIONS:




## Aromatic
- ◯ DIFFUSE
- ◯ INHALE
- ◯ SPRAY BOTTLE
- ◯ _____

## Topical
- ◯ DILLUTE
- ◯ NEAT
- ◯ TEMPLE
- ◯ CHEST
- ◯ STOMACH
- ◯ FEET
- ◯ _____

## Internal
- ◯ ADD TO DRINKING WATER
- ◯ ADD IN FOOD
- ◯ ADD IN CAPSULE
- ◯ UNDER TONGUE
- ◯ _____

NOTES:

# Essential Oil Recipes

NAME: _____

OILS USED: _____

USED FOR: _____
_____

INSTRUCTIONS: _____
_____
_____
_____

## Aromatic
- ○ DIFFUSE
- ○ INHALE
- ○ SPRAY BOTTLE
- ○ _____

## Topical
- ○ DILLUTE
- ○ NEAT
- ○ TEMPLE
- ○ CHEST
- ○ STOMACH
- ○ FEET
- ○ _____

## Internal
- ○ ADD TO DRINKING WATER
- ○ ADD IN FOOD
- ○ ADD IN CAPSULE
- ○ UNDER TONGUE
- ○ _____

NOTES: _____
_____
_____

# Essential Oil Recipes

NAME:

OILS USED:

USED FOR:

INSTRUCTIONS:

## Aromatic
- ○ DIFFUSE
- ○ INHALE
- ○ SPRAY BOTTLE
- ○

## Topical
- ○ DILLUTE
- ○ NEAT
- ○ TEMPLE
- ○ CHEST
- ○ STOMACH
- ○ FEET
- ○

## Internal
- ○ ADD TO DRINKING WATER
- ○ ADD IN FOOD
- ○ ADD IN CAPSULE
- ○ UNDER TONGUE
- ○

NOTES:

# Essential Oil Recipes

NAME: _____

OILS USED: _____

USED FOR: _____
_____

INSTRUCTIONS: _____
_____
_____
_____

## Aromatic
- ○ DIFFUSE
- ○ INHALE
- ○ SPRAY BOTTLE
- ○ _____

## Topical
- ○ DILLUTE
- ○ NEAT
- ○ TEMPLE
- ○ CHEST
- ○ STOMACH
- ○ FEET
- ○ _____

## Internal
- ○ ADD TO DRINKING WATER
- ○ ADD IN FOOD
- ○ ADD IN CAPSULE
- ○ UNDER TONGUE
- ○ _____

NOTES:
_____
_____
_____

# Essential Oil Recipes

NAME:

OILS USED:

USED FOR:

INSTRUCTIONS:

## Aromatic
- ○ DIFFUSE
- ○ INHALE
- ○ SPRAY BOTTLE
- ○ _____

## Topical
- ○ DILLUTE
- ○ NEAT
- ○ TEMPLE
- ○ CHEST
- ○ STOMACH
- ○ FEET
- ○

## Internal
- ○ ADD TO DRINKING WATER
- ○ ADD IN FOOD
- ○ ADD IN CAPSULE
- ○ UNDER TONGUE
- ○ _____

NOTES:

# Essential Oil Recipes

NAME:

OILS USED:

USED FOR:

INSTRUCTIONS:

## Aromatic
- ○ DIFFUSE
- ○ INHALE
- ○ SPRAY BOTTLE
- ○

## Topical
- ○ DILLUTE
- ○ NEAT
- ○ TEMPLE
- ○ CHEST
- ○ STOMACH
- ○ FEET
- ○

## Internal
- ○ ADD TO DRINKING WATER
- ○ ADD IN FOOD
- ○ ADD IN CAPSULE
- ○ UNDER TONGUE
- ○

NOTES:

# Essential Oil Recipes

NAME:

OILS USED:

USED FOR:

INSTRUCTIONS:

## Aromatic
- ○ DIFFUSE
- ○ INHALE
- ○ SPRAY BOTTLE
- ○

## Topical
- ○ DILLUTE
- ○ NEAT
- ○ TEMPLE
- ○ CHEST
- ○ STOMACH
- ○ FEET
- ○

## Internal
- ○ ADD TO DRINKING WATER
- ○ ADD IN FOOD
- ○ ADD IN CAPSULE
- ○ UNDER TONGUE
- ○

NOTES:

# Essential Oil Recipes

NAME: _____

OILS USED: _____

USED FOR: _____
_____

INSTRUCTIONS: _____
_____
_____
_____

## Aromatic
- ◯ DIFFUSE
- ◯ INHALE
- ◯ SPRAY BOTTLE
- ◯ _____

## Topical
- ◯ DILLUTE
- ◯ NEAT
- ◯ TEMPLE
- ◯ CHEST
- ◯ STOMACH
- ◯ FEET
- ◯ _____

## Internal
- ◯ ADD TO DRINKING WATER
- ◯ ADD IN FOOD
- ◯ ADD IN CAPSULE
- ◯ UNDER TONGUE
- ◯ _____

NOTES: _____
_____
_____

# Essential Oil Recipes

NAME:

OILS USED:

USED FOR:

INSTRUCTIONS:

## Aromatic

- ◯ DIFFUSE
- ◯ INHALE
- ◯ SPRAY BOTTLE
- ◯

## Topical

- ◯ DILLUTE
- ◯ NEAT
- ◯ TEMPLE
- ◯ CHEST
- ◯ STOMACH
- ◯ FEET
- ◯

## Internal

- ◯ ADD TO DRINKING WATER
- ◯ ADD IN FOOD
- ◯ ADD IN CAPSULE
- ◯ UNDER TONGUE
- ◯

NOTES:

# Essential Oil Recipes

NAME: _____

OILS USED: _____

USED FOR: _____
_____

INSTRUCTIONS: _____
_____
_____

## Aromatic
- ◯ DIFFUSE
- ◯ INHALE
- ◯ SPRAY BOTTLE
- ◯ _____

## Topical
- ◯ DILLUTE
- ◯ NEAT
- ◯ TEMPLE
- ◯ CHEST
- ◯ STOMACH
- ◯ FEET
- ◯ _____

## Internal
- ◯ ADD TO DRINKING WATER
- ◯ ADD IN FOOD
- ◯ ADD IN CAPSULE
- ◯ UNDER TONGUE
- ◯ _____

NOTES: _____
_____
_____

# Essential Oil Recipes

NAME:

OILS USED:

USED FOR:

INSTRUCTIONS:

## Aromatic
- ○ DIFFUSE
- ○ INHALE
- ○ SPRAY BOTTLE
- ○

## Topical
- ○ DILLUTE
- ○ NEAT
- ○ TEMPLE
- ○ CHEST
- ○ STOMACH
- ○ FEET
- ○

## Internal
- ○ ADD TO DRINKING WATER
- ○ ADD IN FOOD
- ○ ADD IN CAPSULE
- ○ UNDER TONGUE
- ○

NOTES:

# Essential Oil Recipes

NAME:

OILS USED:

USED FOR:

INSTRUCTIONS:

## Aromatic
- ○ DIFFUSE
- ○ INHALE
- ○ SPRAY BOTTLE
- ○ _____

## Topical
- ○ DILLUTE
- ○ NEAT
- ○ TEMPLE
- ○ CHEST
- ○ STOMACH
- ○ FEET
- ○

## Internal
- ○ ADD TO DRINKING WATER
- ○ ADD IN FOOD
- ○ ADD IN CAPSULE
- ○ UNDER TONGUE
- ○ _____

NOTES:

# Essential Oil Recipes

NAME: _____

OILS USED: _____

USED FOR: _____
_____

INSTRUCTIONS: _____
_____
_____
_____

## Aromatic
- ○ DIFFUSE
- ○ INHALE
- ○ SPRAY BOTTLE
- ○ _____

## Topical
- ○ DILLUTE
- ○ NEAT
- ○ TEMPLE
- ○ CHEST
- ○ STOMACH
- ○ FEET
- ○ _____

## Internal
- ○ ADD TO DRINKING WATER
- ○ ADD IN FOOD
- ○ ADD IN CAPSULE
- ○ UNDER TONGUE
- ○ _____

NOTES: _____
_____
_____

# Essential Oil Recipes

NAME:

OILS USED:

USED FOR:

INSTRUCTIONS:

## Aromatic
- ○ DIFFUSE
- ○ INHALE
- ○ SPRAY BOTTLE
- ○ _____

## Topical
- ○ DILLUTE
- ○ NEAT
- ○ TEMPLE
- ○ CHEST
- ○ STOMACH
- ○ FEET
- ○ _____

## Internal
- ○ ADD TO DRINKING WATER
- ○ ADD IN FOOD
- ○ ADD IN CAPSULE
- ○ UNDER TONGUE
- ○ _____

NOTES:

# Essential Oil Recipes

NAME:

OILS USED:

USED FOR:

INSTRUCTIONS:

## Aromatic
- ○ DIFFUSE
- ○ INHALE
- ○ SPRAY BOTTLE
- ○

## Topical
- ○ DILLUTE
- ○ NEAT
- ○ TEMPLE
- ○ CHEST
- ○ STOMACH
- ○ FEET
- ○

## Internal
- ○ ADD TO DRINKING WATER
- ○ ADD IN FOOD
- ○ ADD IN CAPSULE
- ○ UNDER TONGUE
- ○

NOTES:

# Essential Oil Recipes

NAME: _____

OILS USED: _____

USED FOR: _____
_____

INSTRUCTIONS: _____
_____
_____
_____

## Aromatic
- ○ DIFFUSE
- ○ INHALE
- ○ SPRAY BOTTLE
- ○ _____

## Topical
- ○ DILLUTE
- ○ NEAT
- ○ TEMPLE
- ○ CHEST
- ○ STOMACH
- ○ FEET
- ○ _____

## Internal
- ○ ADD TO DRINKING WATER
- ○ ADD IN FOOD
- ○ ADD IN CAPSULE
- ○ UNDER TONGUE
- ○ _____

NOTES: _____
_____
_____

# Essential Oil Recipes

NAME: _____

OILS USED: _____

USED FOR: _____

INSTRUCTIONS: _____

## Aromatic
- ◯ DIFFUSE
- ◯ INHALE
- ◯ SPRAY BOTTLE
- ◯ _____

## Topical
- ◯ DILLUTE
- ◯ NEAT
- ◯ TEMPLE
- ◯ CHEST
- ◯ STOMACH
- ◯ FEET
- ◯ _____

## Internal
- ◯ ADD TO DRINKING WATER
- ◯ ADD IN FOOD
- ◯ ADD IN CAPSULE
- ◯ UNDER TONGUE
- ◯ _____

NOTES: _____

# Essential Oil Recipes

NAME:

OILS USED:

USED FOR:

INSTRUCTIONS:

## Aromatic
- ◯ DIFFUSE
- ◯ INHALE
- ◯ SPRAY BOTTLE
- ◯ _____

## Topical
- ◯ DILLUTE
- ◯ NEAT
- ◯ TEMPLE
- ◯ CHEST
- ◯ STOMACH
- ◯ FEET
- ◯ _____

## Internal
- ◯ ADD TO DRINKING WATER
- ◯ ADD IN FOOD
- ◯ ADD IN CAPSULE
- ◯ UNDER TONGUE
- ◯ _____

NOTES:

# Essential Oil Recipes

NAME: _____

OILS USED: _____

USED FOR: _____
_____

INSTRUCTIONS: _____
_____
_____

## Aromatic
- ◯ DIFFUSE
- ◯ INHALE
- ◯ SPRAY BOTTLE
- ◯ _____

## Topical
- ◯ DILLUTE
- ◯ NEAT
- ◯ TEMPLE
- ◯ CHEST
- ◯ STOMACH
- ◯ FEET
- ◯ _____

## Internal
- ◯ ADD TO DRINKING WATER
- ◯ ADD IN FOOD
- ◯ ADD IN CAPSULE
- ◯ UNDER TONGUE
- ◯ _____

NOTES: _____
_____
_____

# Essential Oil Recipes

NAME:

OILS USED:

USED FOR:

INSTRUCTIONS:

## Aromatic
- ○ DIFFUSE
- ○ INHALE
- ○ SPRAY BOTTLE
- ○ _____

## Topical
- ○ DILLUTE
- ○ NEAT
- ○ TEMPLE
- ○ CHEST
- ○ STOMACH
- ○ FEET
- ○ _____

## Internal
- ○ ADD TO DRINKING WATER
- ○ ADD IN FOOD
- ○ ADD IN CAPSULE
- ○ UNDER TONGUE
- ○ _____

NOTES:

# Essential Oil Recipes

NAME:

OILS USED:

USED FOR:

INSTRUCTIONS:

## Aromatic
- ○ DIFFUSE
- ○ INHALE
- ○ SPRAY BOTTLE
- ○

## Topical
- ○ DILLUTE
- ○ NEAT
- ○ TEMPLE
- ○ CHEST
- ○ STOMACH
- ○ FEET
- ○

## Internal
- ○ ADD TO DRINKING WATER
- ○ ADD IN FOOD
- ○ ADD IN CAPSULE
- ○ UNDER TONGUE
- ○

NOTES:

# Essential Oil Recipes

NAME: _____

OILS USED: _____

USED FOR: _____
_____

INSTRUCTIONS: _____
_____
_____
_____

## Aromatic
- ◯ DIFFUSE
- ◯ INHALE
- ◯ SPRAY BOTTLE
- ◯ _____

## Topical
- ◯ DILLUTE
- ◯ NEAT
- ◯ TEMPLE
- ◯ CHEST
- ◯ STOMACH
- ◯ FEET
- ◯

## Internal
- ◯ ADD TO DRINKING WATER
- ◯ ADD IN FOOD
- ◯ ADD IN CAPSULE
- ◯ UNDER TONGUE
- ◯ _____

NOTES: _____
_____
_____

# Essential Oil Recipes

NAME:

OILS USED:

USED FOR:

INSTRUCTIONS:

## Aromatic
- ◯ DIFFUSE
- ◯ INHALE
- ◯ SPRAY BOTTLE
- ◯

## Topical
- ◯ DILLUTE
- ◯ NEAT
- ◯ TEMPLE
- ◯ CHEST
- ◯ STOMACH
- ◯ FEET
- ◯

## Internal
- ◯ ADD TO DRINKING WATER
- ◯ ADD IN FOOD
- ◯ ADD IN CAPSULE
- ◯ UNDER TONGUE
- ◯

NOTES:

# Essential Oil Recipes

NAME:

OILS USED:

USED FOR:

INSTRUCTIONS:

## Aromatic
- ◯ DIFFUSE
- ◯ INHALE
- ◯ SPRAY BOTTLE
- ◯

## Topical
- ◯ DILLUTE
- ◯ NEAT
- ◯ TEMPLE
- ◯ CHEST
- ◯ STOMACH
- ◯ FEET
- ◯

## Internal
- ◯ ADD TO DRINKING WATER
- ◯ ADD IN FOOD
- ◯ ADD IN CAPSULE
- ◯ UNDER TONGUE
- ◯

NOTES:

# Essential Oil Recipes

NAME: _____

OILS USED: _____

USED FOR: _____
_____

INSTRUCTIONS: _____
_____
_____
_____

### Aromatic
- ○ DIFFUSE
- ○ INHALE
- ○ SPRAY BOTTLE
- ○ _____

### Topical
- ○ DILLUTE
- ○ NEAT
- ○ TEMPLE
- ○ CHEST
- ○ STOMACH
- ○ FEET
- ○ _____

### Internal
- ○ ADD TO DRINKING WATER
- ○ ADD IN FOOD
- ○ ADD IN CAPSULE
- ○ UNDER TONGUE
- ○ _____

NOTES: _____
_____
_____

# Essential Oil Recipes

NAME: _____

OILS USED: _____

USED FOR: _____
_____

INSTRUCTIONS: _____
_____
_____
_____

## Aromatic
- ◯ DIFFUSE
- ◯ INHALE
- ◯ SPRAY BOTTLE
- ◯ _____

## Topical
- ◯ DILLUTE
- ◯ NEAT
- ◯ TEMPLE
- ◯ CHEST
- ◯ STOMACH
- ◯ FEET
- ◯ _____

## Internal
- ◯ ADD TO DRINKING WATER
- ◯ ADD IN FOOD
- ◯ ADD IN CAPSULE
- ◯ UNDER TONGUE
- ◯ _____

NOTES: _____
_____
_____

# Diffuser Blends

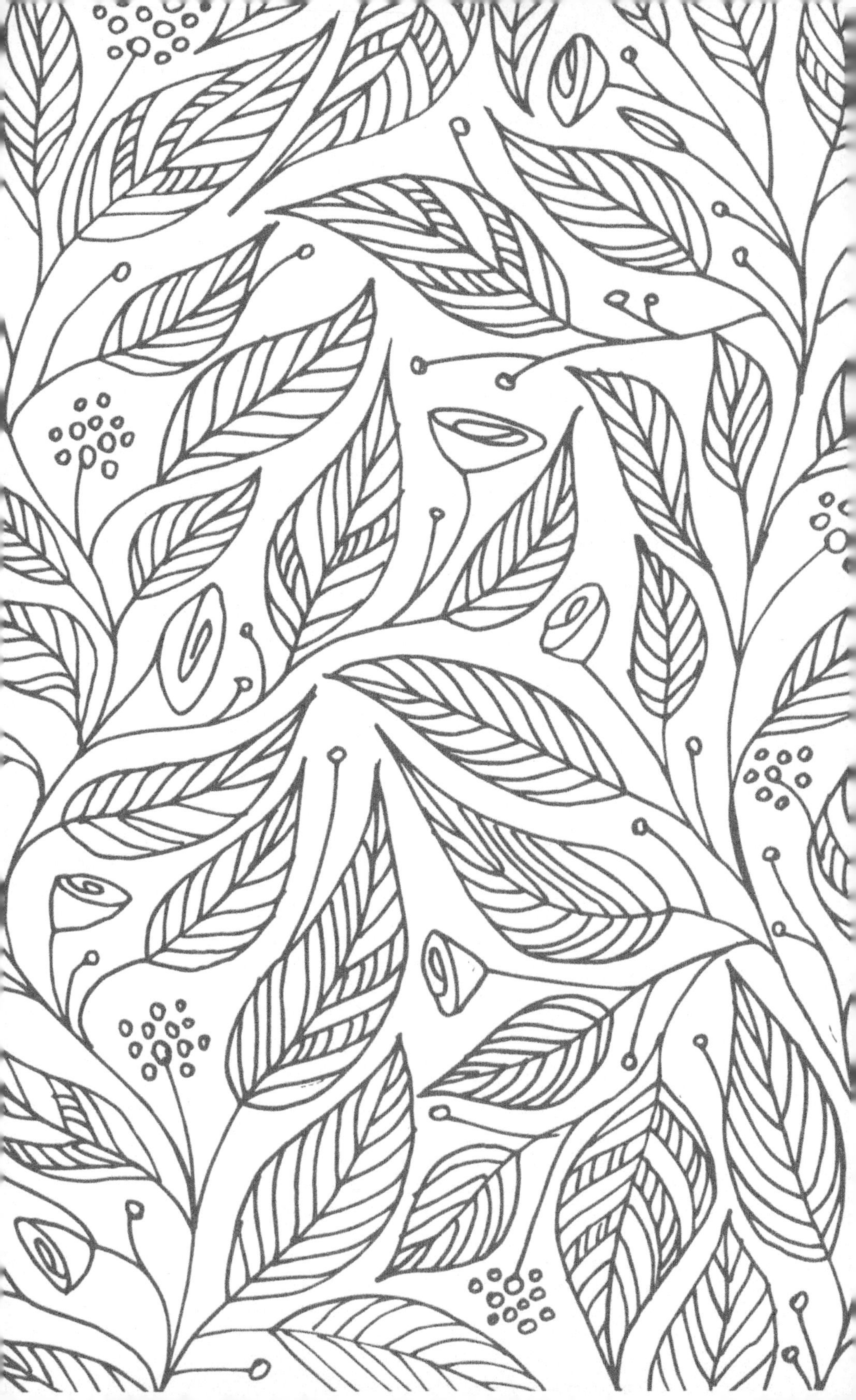

# Lavender Blends

## DIFFUSER BLENDS

### Sea Breeze

2 DROPS LAVENDER

3 DROPS LIME

1 DROP SPEARMINT

### Ocean Breeze

4 DROPS LAVENDER

3 DROPS ROSEMARY

2 DROPS LEMONGRASS

### Cool Down

4 DROPS SPEARMINT

2 DROPS LAVENDER

2 DROPS PEPPERMINT

### Lavender Mint

4 DROPS LAVENDER

3 DROPS PEPPERMINT

1 DROP VETIVER

### Peacefulness

3 DROPS LAVENDER

3 DROPS VETIVER

2 DROPS YLANG YLANG

### Clean Air

3 DROPS LAVENDER

3 DROPS TANGERINE

3 DROPS EUCALYPTUS

### Creative Spark

3 DROPS LAVENDER

3 DROPS SWEET ORANGE

1 DROP PEPPERMINT

### Mindfulness

2 DROPS LAVENDER

3 DROPS BERGAMOT

2 DROPS ROSEMARY

**NOTES:**

# Wellness Blends

**DIFFUSER BLENDS**

### Energizing

4 DROPS PEPPERMINT

4 DROPS CINNAMON

2 DROPS ROSEMARY

### Extreme Focus

4 DROPS BALANCE

2 DROPS FRANKINCENSE

2 DROPS VETIVER

### Inner Calm

3 DROPS ELEVATION

3 DROPS BERGAMOT

3 DROPS FRANKINCENSE

### Tranquility

3 DROPS LAVENDER

2 DROPS LIME

3 DROPS MANDARIN

### Lover of Life

3 DROPS ROSEMARY

3 DROPS PEPPERMINT

3 DROPS FRANKINCENSE

### Stress Be Gone

3 DROPS LAVENDER

2 DROPS CHAMOMILE

2 DROPS YLANG YLANG

### Relaxation

3 DROPS BERGAMOT

3 DROPS PATCHOULI

3 DROPS YLANG YLANG

### Active Life

2 DROPS GRAPEFRUIT

3 DROPS PEPPERMINT

3 DROPS ROSEMARY

**NOTES:**

# Happiness Blends

**DIFFUSER BLENDS**

### Cheerful

3 DROPS WILD ORANGE

3 DROPS FRANKINCENSE

1 DROP CINNAMON

### Sweetness

3 DROPS BERGAMOT

2 DROPS GERANIUM

3 DROPS LAVENDER

### Inner Peace

2 DROPS PEPPERMINT

2 DROPS LAVENDER

2 DROPS WILD ORANGE

### Zoned Out

2 DROPS ROSEMARY

2 DROPS CINNAMON

1 DROP CLOVE

### With Purpose

3 DROPS LEMON

2 DROPS OREGANO

2 DROPS ON GUARD

### Laughter

3 DROPS LEMON

3 DROPS TANGERINE

2 DROPS MELALEUCA

### Booster

2 DROPS LAVENDER

3 DROPS SWEET ORANGE

3 DROPS PEPPERMINT

### Mindfulness

3 DROPS LAVENDER

3 DROPS BERGAMOT

1 DROP CLOVE

**NOTES:**

# Well Rested Blends

## DIFFUSER BLENDS

### Well Rested
3 DROPS JUNIPER BERRY

3 DROPS CHAMOMILE

3 DROPS LAVENDER

### Well Rested 2
4 DROPS CEDARWOOD

3 DROPS LAVENDER

1 DROP VETIVER

### Well Rested 3
2 DROPS FRANKINCENSE

3 DROPS VETIVER

2 DROPS LAVENDER

### Well Rested 4
3 DROPS BALANCE

2 DROPS LAVENDER

2 DROPS CHAMOMILE

### Well Rested 5
3 DROPS LAVENDER

2 DROPS MARJORAM

2 DROPS ORANGE

### Well Rested 6
3 DROPS LEMON

3 DROPS LAVENDER

2 DROPS PEPPERMINT

### Well Rested 7
5 DROPS PEPPERMINT

4 DROPS EUCALYPTUS

2 DROPS MYRRH

### Well Rested 8
3 DROPS LAVENDER

3 DROPS CHAMOMILE

1 DROP CLOVE

**NOTES:**

# Clean House Blends

## DIFFUSER BLENDS

### Sparkly Clean
3 DROPS LEMON

3 DROPS PEPPERMINT

3 DROPS EUCALYPTUS

### Decluttering
4 DROPS LEMON

3 DROPS LEMONGRASS

2 DROPS PEPPERMINT

### Nice & Tidy
3 DROPS EUCALYPTUS

3 DROPS WILD ORANGE

3 DROPS LIME

### Spring Cleaning
4 DROPS LEMON

3 DROPS LAVENDER

2 DROPS ROSEMARY

### Fresh Scent
3 DROPS LEMON

3 DROPS EASY AIR

3 DROPS LIME

### Glossy Clean
4 DROPS FRANKINCENSE

4 DROPS CYPRESS

2 DROPS YLANG YLANG

### Tidy Home
1 DROP ROSE

1 DROP CARDAMOM

2 DROPS WILD ORANGE

### Housekeeper
2 DROPS CINNAMON

2 DROPS CARDAMOM

2 DROPS LEMOM

**NOTES:**

# Personality Blends

**DIFFUSER BLENDS**

### Confident

2 DROPS SPEARMINT

2 DROPS TANGERINE

2 DROPS BERGAMOT

### Carefree

5 DROPS BERGAMOT

2 DROPS PATCHOULI

2 DROPS LIME

### Happy

2 DROPS WILD ORANGE

2 DROPS GRAPEFRUIT

2 DROPS CLOVE

### Inspired

1 DROP ROSE

1 DROP PURIFY

2 DROPS JUNIPER BERRY

### Focused

3 DROPS DOUGLAS FIR

2 DROPS LEMON

1 DROP PEPPERMINT

### Energetic

2 DROPS PEPPERMINT

3 DROPS GRAPEFRUIT

3 DROPS BERGAMOT

### Motivated

2 DROPS ELEVATION

2 DROPS CYPRESS

2 DROPS LIME

### Peaceful

2 DROPS FRANKINCENSE

2 DROPS WHITE FIR

2 DROPS LAVENDER

**NOTES:**

# Day to Day Blends

## DIFFUSER BLENDS

### SLEEP TIME

4 DROPS LAVENDER

4 DROPS CEDARWOOD

3 DROPS CHAMOMILE

### Combat Nausea

3 DROPS GINGER

5 DROPS PEPPERMINT

1 DROP BALANCE

### Anti-Stress

4 DROPS BERGAMOT

4 DROPS FRANKINCENSE

1 DROP PEPPERMINT

### Headaches

2 DROPS FRANKINCENSE

2 DROPS LAVENDER

4 DROPS PEPPERMINT

### Allergy Be Gone

3 DROPS LAVENDER

3 DROPS LEMON

3 DROPS PEPPERMINT

### Breathe Easy

4 DROPS PEPPERMINT

2 DROPS EUCALYPTUS

2 DROPS LEMON

### Concentration

4 DROPS LAVENDER

4 DROPS MELALEUCA

4 DROPS FRANKINCENSE

### Immune Boost

2 DROPS FRANKINCENSE

5 DROPS LEMON

2 DROPS PEPPERMINT

**NOTES:**

# Spring Blends

## DIFFUSER BLENDS

### Welcome Spring

2 DROPS GERANIUM

2 DROPS LEMON

2 DROPS GRAPEFRUIT

### Spring Garden

2 DROPS BASIL

2 DROPS PEPPERMINT

2 DROPS LIME

### Fresh & Clean

4 DROPS GRAPEFRUIT

3 DROPS PEPPERMINT

3 DROPS CLARY SAGE

### Fresh Flowers

5 DROPS CLARY SAGE

3 DROPS LAVENDAR

2 DROPS GERANIUM

### Spring Petals

2 DROPS YLANG YLANG

2 DROPS PEPPERMINT

2 DROPS JADE LEMON

### Mother Nature

3 DROPS PEPPERMINT

3 DROPS LAVENDAR

3 DROPS LEMON

### Spring Cleaning

2 DROPS LAVENDAR

3 DROPS LEMON

3 DROPS ROSEMARY

### Good Morning

4 DROPS JOY

3 DROPS LEMON

1 DROP TANGERINE

**NOTES:**

# Summer Blends

**DIFFUSER BLENDS**

### Sweet Sunshine

3 DROPS LEMONGRASS

2 DROPS ORANGE

1 DROP PEPPERMINT

### Summer Loving

2 DROPS JUNIPER BERRY

2 DROPS GRAPEFRUIT

2 DROPS WILD ORANGE

### Sunny Days

3 DROPS TANGERINE

3 DROPS LEMON

1 DROP PEPPERMINT

### Ocean Breeze

3 DROPS BERGAMOT

3 DROPS LAVENDER

3 DROPS ROSEMARY

### Hammock Time

2 DROPS LAVENDER

2 DROPS CEDARWOOD

2 DROPS WILD ORANGE

### Beach Memories

2 DROPS SPEARMINT

3 DROPS TANGERINE

2 DROPS BERGAMOT

### Citrus Twist

2 DROPS TANGERINE

2 DROPS GRAPEFRUIT

2 DROPS LEMON

### Sun Kissed

2 DROPS TEA TREE

2 DROPS LEMON

2 DROPS LIME

**NOTES:**

# Autumn Blends

**DIFFUSER BLENDS**

## Pumpkin Spice

5 DROPS CINNAMON

2 DROPS NUTMEG

3 DROPS CLOVE

## Cider

4 DROPS ORANGE

3 DROPS CINNAMON

3 DROPS GINGER

## Snickerdoodle

5 DROPS STRESS AWAY

3 DROPS CINNAMON

2 DROPS NUTMEG

## Changing Leaves

5 DROPS CLOVE

5 DROPS CEDARWOOD

5 DROPS ORANGE

## Flannel Sheets

5 DROPS BLACK SPRUCE

4 DROPS STRESS AWAY

4 DROPS ORANGE

## Giving Thanks

5 DROPS CINNAMON

3 DROPS ORANGE

2 DROPS NUTMEG

## Sweater Weather

5 DROPS ORANGE

4 DROPS THIEVES

1 DROP GINGER

## Autumn Breeze

5 DROPS CHRISTMAS SPIRIT

2 DROPS CLOVE

1 DROP LEMON

**NOTES:**

# Winter Blends

**DIFFUSER BLENDS**

### Winter Citrus

2 DROPS PEPPERMINT

2 DROPS LEMONGRASS

2 DROPS TANGERINE

### Snow Days

2 DROPS STRESS AWAY

2 DROPS THIEVES

2 DROPS CITRUS

### Classic Winter

2 DROPS CEDARWOOD

2 DROPS LAVENDER

2 DROPS ROSEMARY

### Cozy Home

2 DROPS BERGAMOT

2 DROPS ORANGE

2 DROPS THIEVES

### Snowflake

2 DROPS LAVENDER

2 DROPS LEMON

2 DROPS DIGIZE

### Mother Nature

3 DROPS PEPPERMINT

3 DROPS LAVENDER

3 DROPS LEMON

### Holiday Baking

2 DROPS CASSIA

2 DROPS VETIVER

2 DROPS LAVENDAR

### Winter Memories

2 DROPS BERGAMOT

2 DROPS WILD ORANGE

2 DROPS EUCALYPTUS

**NOTES:**

# Holiday Blends

**DIFFUSER BLENDS**

### Deck The Halls

4 DROPS PINE

2 DROPS BLUE SPRUCE

2 DROPS CEDARWOOD

### Snow Angels

4 DROPS STRESS AWAY

3 FRESH CITRUS

1 DROP FRANKINCENSE

### Candy Cane

4 DROPS PEPPERMINT

3 DROPS BERGAMOT

1 DROP WILD ORANGE

### Spiced Cider

3 DROPS WILD ORANGE

2 DROPS CINNAMON BARK

1 DROP CLOVE

### Sugar Plum Fairy

3 DROPS CITRUS BLISS

2 DROPS DOUGLAS FIR

2 DROPS MOTIVATE

### Merry & Bright

3 DROPS LEMON

2 DROPS DOUGLAS FIR

2 DROPS CINNAMON

### Oh, Holy Night

5 DROPS THIEVES

2 DROPS FRANKINCENSE

2 DROPS CITRUS FRESH

### Gingerbread Man

4 DROPS GINGER

2 DROPS CLOVES

2 DROPS CINNAMON

**NOTES:**

# Notes

# Notes

# Notes

# Notes

# Notes

# Notes

Made in the USA
Monee, IL
22 July 2020